Plant Based Essential Recipes

50 Delicious Plant Based Recipes for Tasty Meals

Tanya Lang

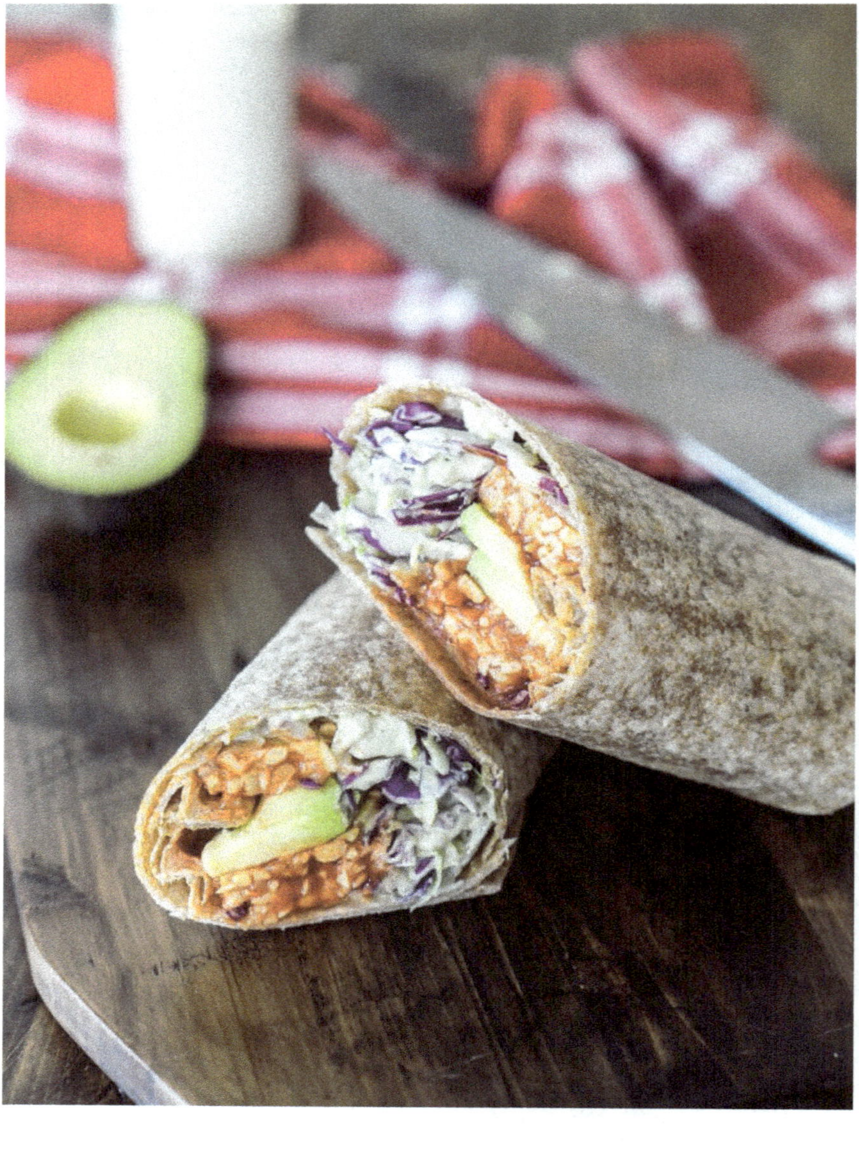

TABLE OF CONTENT

Quinoa Cherry Tortilla Wraps

• Preparation Time: 15-30 minutes | Cooking Time: 25 minutes | Servings: 4

Ingredients:

- ½ cup brown quinoa
- Salt and black pepper to taste
- 2 tsp olive oil
- 1 ½ cups shredded carrots
- 1 ¼ cups fresh cherries, pitted and halved
- 4 scallions, chopped
- 2 tbsp plain vinegar
- 2 tbsp low-sodium soy sauce
- 1 tbsp pure maple syrup
- 4 (8-inch) tortilla wraps

Directions:

• Cook the quinoa in 1 cup of slightly salted water in a medium pot over medium heat until tender and the water absorbs, 10 minutes. Fluff and set aside to warm.

- Heat the olive oil in a medium skillet and sauté

the carrots, cherries, and scallions. While cooking, in a small bowl, mix the vinegar, soy sauce, and maple syrup. Stir the mixture into the vegetable mixture. Simmer for 5 minutes and turn the heat off.

- Spread the tortillas on a flat surface, spoon the mixture at the center, fold the sides and ends to wrap in the filling.
- Serve warm.

Nutrition:

- Calories 282 kcal Fats 6. 5g Carbs 48g Protein 8. 3g

Quinoa With Mixed Herbs

• Preparation Time: 15-30 minutes | Cooking Time: 20 minutes | Servings: 4 Ingredients:

- 1 cup quinoa, well-rinsed
- 2 cups vegetable broth
- Salt to taste
- 2 garlic cloves, minced, divided
- ¼ cup chopped chives
- 2 tbsp finely chopped parsley
- 2 tbsp finely chopped basil
- 2 tbsp finely chopped mint
- 2 tbsp finely chopped soft sundried tomatoes
- 1 tbsp olive oil (optional)
- ½ tsp lemon zest
- 1 tbsp fresh lemon juice
- 2 tbsp minced walnuts
- Salt and black pepper to taste

Directions:

- In a medium pot, combine the quinoa, vegetable broth, ¼ tsp of salt, and half of the garlic in a medium saucepan. Boil until the quinoa is tender and the liquid absorbs, 10-15 minutes. • Open the lid, fluff with a fork, and stir in the chives, parsley, basil, mint, tomatoes, olive oil,

zest, lemon juice, and walnuts. Warm for 5 minutes.

- Dish the food and serve warm.

Nutrition:

- Calories 393 kcal Fats 17. 1g Carbs 31. 9g Protein 27. 8g

Chickpea Avocado Pizza

• Preparation Time: 15-30 minutes | Cooking Time: 40 minutes | Servings: 4

Ingredients:

- For the pizza crust:
- 3 ½ cups whole-wheat flour
- 1 tsp yeast
- 1 tsp salt
- 1 pinch sugar
- 3 tbsp olive oil
- 1 cup of warm water
- For the topping:
- 1 cup red pizza sauce
- 1 cup baby spinach
- Salt and black pepper to taste
- 1 (15 oz) can chickpeas, drained and rinsed
- 1 medium avocado, pitted, peeled, and chopped
- ¼ cup grated plant-based Parmesan cheese

Directions:

- Preheat the oven the 350 F and lightly grease a pizza pan with cooking spray.

- In a medium bowl, mix the flour, nutritional yeast, salt, sugar, olive oil, and warm water until smooth dough forms. Allow rising for an hour or until the dough doubles in size.
- Spread the dough on the pizza pan and apply the pizza sauce on top.
- Top with the spinach, chickpeas, avocado, and plant Parmesan cheese.
- Bake the pizza for 20 minutes or until the cheese melts.
- Remove from the oven, cool for 5 minutes, slice, and serve.

Nutrition:

- Calories 678 kcal Fats 22. 7g Carbs 104. 1g Protein 23. 5g

White Bean Stuffed Squash

• Preparation Time: 15-30 minutes | Cooking Time: 60 minutes | Servings: 4

Ingredients:

- 2 pounds large acorn squash
- 2 tbsp olive oil
- 3 garlic cloves, minced
- 1 (15 oz) can white beans, drained and rinsed
- 1 cup chopped spinach leaves
- ½ cup vegetable stock
- Salt and black pepper to taste
- ½ tsp cumin powder
- ½ tsp chili powder

Directions:

- Preheat the oven to 350 F.
- Cut the squash into half and scoop out the seeds.
- Season with salt and pepper and place face down on a sheet pan. Bake for 45 minutes. • While the squash cooks, heat the olive oil in a medium pot over medium

heat. • Sauté the garlic until fragrant, 30 seconds, and mix in the beans. Cook for 1 minute. • Stir in the spinach, allow wilting for 2 minutes, and season with salt, black pepper, cumin

powder, and chili powder. Cook for 2 minutes and turn the heat off.

- When the squash is fork-tender, remove it from the oven and fill the holes with the bean and spinach mixture.
- Serve warm.

Nutrition:

- Calories 365 kcal Fats 34. 6g Carbs 16. 7g Protein 2. 3g

Grilled Zucchini And Spinach Pizza

• Preparation Time: 15-30 minutes | Cooking Time: 30 minutes | Servings: 4

Ingredients:

- For the pizza crust:
- 3 ½ cups whole-wheat flour
- 1 tsp yeast
- 1 tsp salt
- 1 pinch sugar
- 3 tbsp olive oil
- 1 cup of warm water
- For the topping:
- 1 cup marinara sauce
- 2 large zucchinis, sliced
- ½ cup chopped spinach
- ¼ cup pitted and sliced black olives
- ½ cup grated plant Parmesan cheese

Directions:

• Preheat the oven the 350 F and lightly grease a pizza pan with cooking spray. • In a medium bowl, mix the flour, nutritional yeast, salt, sugar, olive oil, and warm water until

smooth dough forms. Allow rising for an hour or until the dough doubles in size. Spread the dough on the pizza pan and apply the pizza sauce on top.

- Meanwhile, heat a grill pan over medium heat, season the zucchinis with salt, black pepper, and cook in the pan until slightly charred on both sides.
- Set the cucumbers on the pizza crust and top with the spinach, olives, and plant Parmesan cheese. Bake the pizza for 20 minutes or until the cheese melts. Remove from the oven, cool for 5 minutes, slice, and serve.

Nutrition:

- Calories 519 kcal Fats 13. 4g Carbs 87. 5g Protein 19. 6g

Honey-Almond Popcorn

Preparation Time: 5 minutes | Cooking Time: 10 minutes | Servings: 4

Ingredients:

- 1/2 cup popcorn kernels
- 2 tablespoons honey
- 1/2 teaspoon sea salt
- 2 tablespoons coconut sugar
- 1 cup roasted almonds
- 1/4 cup walnut oil

Directions:

- Take a pot, place it over medium-low heat, add oil and when it melts, add four kernels and wait until they sizzle.
- Then add the remaining kernel, toss until coated, sprinkle with sugar, drizzle with honey, shut the pot with the lid, and shake the kernels until popped completely, adding almonds halfway.
- Once all the kernels have popped, season them with salt and serve straight away.

Nutrition:

- Calories: 120 Cal Fat: 4.5 g Carbs: 19 g Protein: 1 g Fiber: 1 g

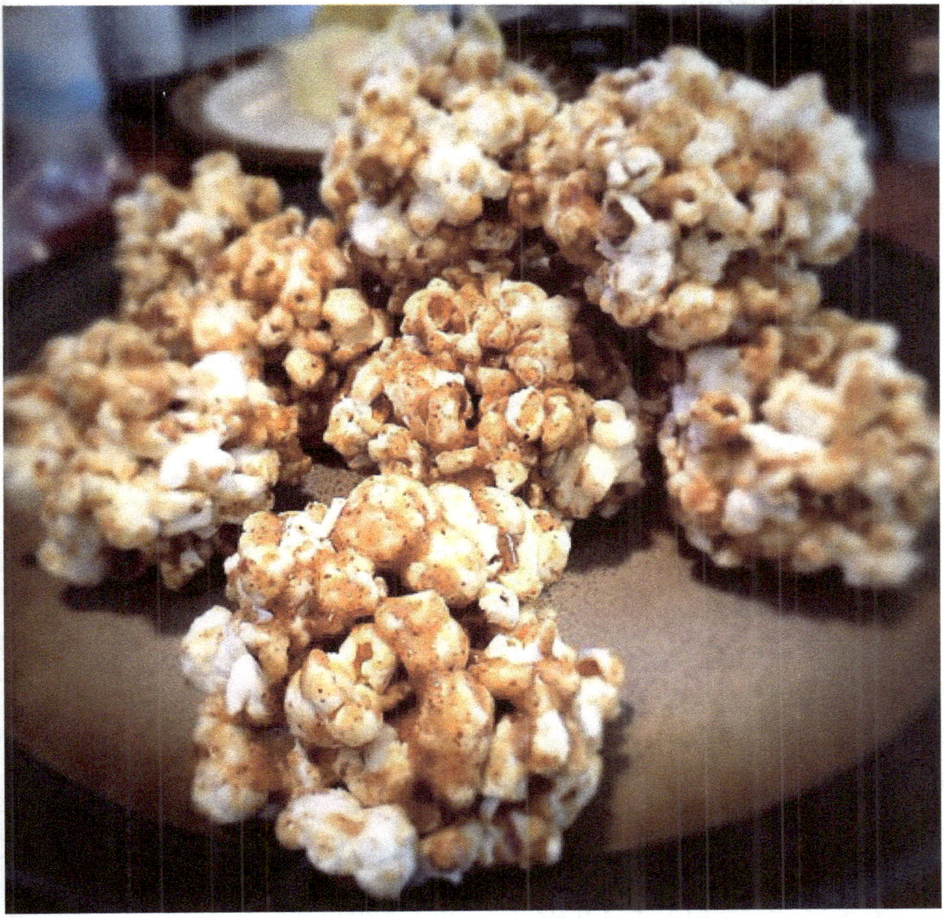

Turmeric Snack Bites

Preparation Time: 35 minutes | Cooking Time: 0 minute | Servings: 10

Ingredients:

- 1 cup Medjool dates, pitted, chopped
- 1/2 cup walnuts
- 1 teaspoon ground turmeric
- 1 tablespoon cocoa powder, unsweetened
- 1/2 teaspoon ground cinnamon
- 1/2 cup shredded coconut, unsweetened

Directions:

- Place all the ingredients in a food processor and pulse for 2 minutes until a smooth mixture comes together.
- Tip the mixture in a bowl and then shape it into ten small balls, 1 tablespoon of the mixture per ball and then refrigerate for 30 minutes.
- Serve straight away.

Nutrition:

- Calories: 109 Cal Fat: 2 g Carbs: 13 g Protein: 1 g Fiber: 0 g

Watermelon Pizza

Preparation Time: 10 minutes | Cooking Time: 0 minute | Servings: 10

Ingredients:

- 1/2 cup strawberries, halved
- 1/2 cup blueberries
- 1 watermelon
- 1/2 cup raspberries
- 1 cup of coconut yogurt
- 1/2 cup pomegranate seeds
- 1/2 cup cherries
- Maple syrup as needed

Directions:

- Cut watermelon into 3-inch thick slices, then spread yogurt on one side, leaving some space in the edges, and then top evenly with fruits and drizzle with maple syrup.
- Cut the watermelon into wedges and then serve.

Nutrition:

- Calories: 150 Cal Fat: 4 g Carbs: 21 g Protein: 10 g Fiber: 2 g

Nooch Popcorn

• Preparation Time: 10 minutes | Cooking Time: 10 minutes | Servings: 4

Ingredients:

- 1/3 cup nutritional yeast
- 1 teaspoon of sea salt
- 3 tablespoons coconut oil
- ½ cup popcorn kernels

Directions:

- Place yeast in a large bowl, stir in salt and set aside until required.
- Take a medium saucepan, place it over medium-high heat, add oil and when it melts, add

four kernels and wait until they sizzle.

- Then add the remaining kernel, toss until coated, shut the pan with the lid, and shake the kernels until popped completely.
- When done, transfer popcorn to the yeast mixture, shut with lid, and shape well until coated. • Serve straight away

Nutrition:

- Calories: 160 Cal Fat: 6 g Carbs: 28 g Protein: 3 g Fiber: 4 g

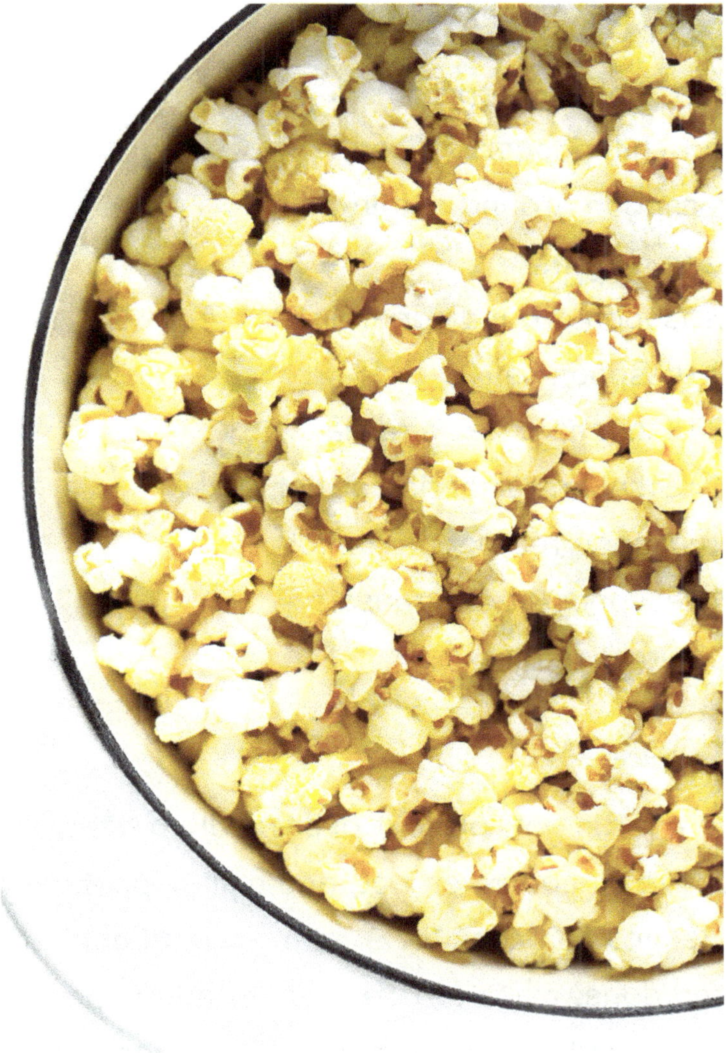

Masala Popcorn

Preparation Time: 5 minutes | Cooking Time: 15 minutes | Servings: 4

Ingredients:

- 3 cups popped popcorn
- 2 hot chili peppers, sliced
- 1 teaspoon ground cumin
- 6 curry leaves
- 1 teaspoon ground coriander
- 1/3 teaspoon salt
- 1/8 teaspoon chaat masala
- 1/4 teaspoon turmeric powder
- ¼ teaspoon red pepper flakes
- 1/4 teaspoon garam masala
- 1/3 cup olive oil

Directions:

- Take a large pot, place it over medium heat, add half of the oil and when hot, add chili peppers and curry leaves and cook for 3 minutes until golden.
- When done, transfer curry leaves and pepper to a plate lined with paper towels and set aside until required.

- Add remaining oil into the pot, add remaining ingredients except for popcorns, stir until mixed and cook for 1 minute until fragrant.
- Then tip in popcorns, remove the pan from heat, stir well until coated, and then sprinkle with bay leaves and red chili.
- Toss until mixed and serve straight away.

Nutrition:

- Calories: 150 Cal Fat: 9 g Carbs: 15 g Protein: 2 g Fiber: 4 g

Cauliflower Nuggets

Preparation Time: 35 minutes | Cooking Time: 0 minutes | Servings: 4

Ingredients:

- 3 tablespoon yeast flakes
- 60 ml of soy milk
- ½ cauliflower
- 2 tablespoons of oil
- ½ cup breadcrumbs
- 30 g flour
- Salt and pepper

Directions:

- Separate the cauliflower into florets and wash.
- Mix the flour, yeast flakes, milk, salt, and pepper.
- Roll the cauliflower in the mass and then roll in breadcrumbs.
- Place on a baking sheet and drizzle with oil.
- Bake for about 35 minutes at 200 degrees Celsius, until the cauliflower is cooked through.

Nutrition:

- Calories: 279 Fat: 15.4g Carbs: 20.5g Protein:

12.1g Fiber: 3.2g

Cauliflower Potato Burgers

Preparation Time: 15 minutes | Cooking Time: 7 minutes | Servings: 2

Ingredients:

- 7 oz cauliflower rice
- 1/4 cup mashed potato
- 1 tablespoon almond flour
- 1 teaspoon salt
- 1 teaspoon white pepper
- 1 tablespoon coconut yogurt
- 1 tablespoon breadcrumbs
- 1/2 cup water, for cooking

Directions:

- In the mixing bowl combine cauliflower rice and mashed potato.
- Add almond flour, salt, white pepper, and coconut yogurt.
- Then wear gloves and make medium size burgers from the mixture.
- Sprinkle every burger with breadcrumbs and wrap it in the foil.

- Pour water into the instant pot bowl and insert the steamer rack.
- Place wrapped burgers on the steamer rack and close the lid.
- Cook the meal on High (Manual mode) for 7 minutes. Then allow natural pressure release for

10 minutes.

Nutrition:

- Calories: 163, Fat: 9, Fiber: 4.8, Carbs: 17, Protein: 6.6

Sweet Potato Burgers

• Preparation Time: 10 minutes | Cooking Time: 20 minutes | Servings: 2

Ingredients:

- 1 sweet potato
- 1/2 onion, diced
- 1 teaspoon chives
- 1/2 teaspoon salt
- 1 teaspoon cayenne pepper
- 3 tablespoon flax meal
- 1/2 cup kale
- 1 teaspoon olive oil
- 1/2 cup water, for cooking

Directions:

- Pour water into the instant pot and insert the steamer rack.
- Place sweet potato on the steamer rack and close the lid.
- Cook the vegetables on Manual mode (High pressure) for 15 minutes (quick pressure

release).

• Meanwhile, place onion, chives, and kale in the blender. Blend until smooth. • Transfer the blended mixture to the mixing bowl.

• When the sweet potato is cooked – cut it into halves and scoop all the flesh into the kale

mixture. Mix it up carefully with the help of the fork.

• Add flax meal, salt, and cayenne pepper. Stir well.

• With the help of the fingertips make medium burgers.

• Clean the instant pot bowl and put olive oil inside.

• Preheat for 2-3 minutes on Sauté mode.

• Then add burgers and cook them for 2 minutes from each side on Sauté mode.

Nutrition:

• Calories: 139, Fat: 6.4, Fiber: 6, Carbs: 19.7, Protein: 4.3

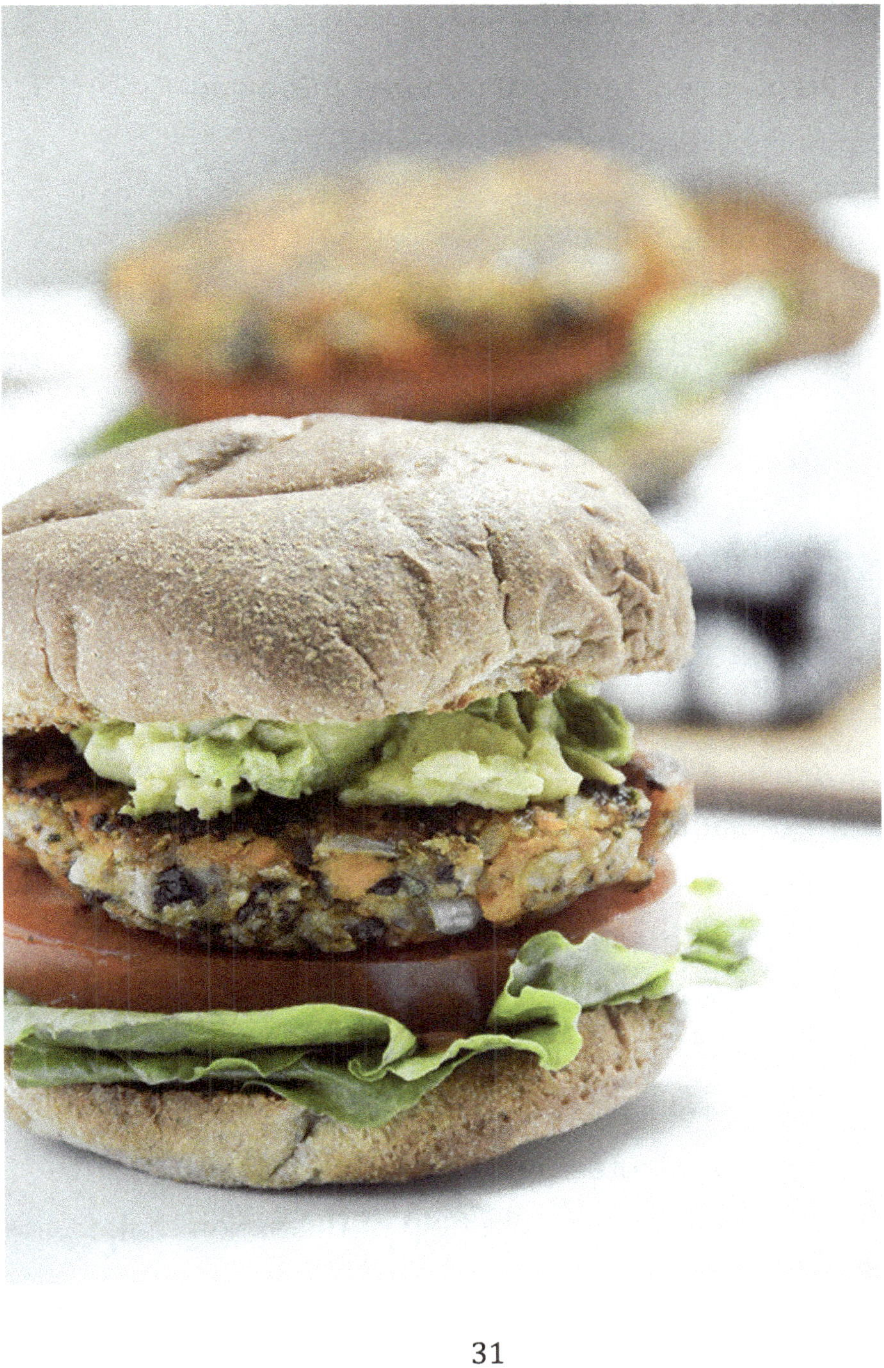

Potato Patties

• Preparation Time: 10 minutes | Cooking Time: 15 minutes | Servings: 4

Ingredients:

- 3 russet potatoes, peeled
- 3 tablespoon aquafaba
- 1/2 teaspoon salt
- 1 teaspoon almond butter
- 1/2 teaspoon smoked paprika
- 1/4 teaspoon chili flakes
- 2 tablespoon wheat flour

Directions:

• With the help of the hand mixer, whisk aquafaba until you get soft peaks.

• Then grate potatoes and combine them with aquafaba in the mixing bowl.

• Add salt, smoked paprika, chili flakes, and wheat flour. Mix it up carefully. • Preheat the instant pot on Sauté mode for 4 minutes. Add almond butter and melt it.

• Then with the help of the spoon make

medium patties; press them a little with the help of

hand palms and put in the hot almond butter.

- Cook the patties for 3 minutes then flip into another side. Cook the patties for 4 minutes more.

Nutrition:

- Calories: 150, Fat: 2.5, Fiber: 4.4, Carbs: 29, Protein: 4

Lentil Burgers

• Preparation Time: 20 minutes | Cooking Time: 26 minutes | Servings: 7

Ingredients:

- 1 cup lentils, soaked overnight
- 1 cup of water
- 1/2 carrot, peeled
- 1 teaspoon cayenne pepper
- 4 tablespoon wheat flour
- 1 teaspoon salt
- 1 teaspoon olive oil
- 1 tablespoon dried dill

Directions:

• Put lentils in the Instant pot together with water, carrot, salt, and cayenne pepper. • Close the lid and set Manual mode (High pressure).

• Cook the ingredients for 25 minutes and allow natural pressure release for 10 minutes. • Transfer the cooked ingredients in the blender and blend until smooth.

• Add wheat flour and dried dill. Mix it up

until smooth. If the mixture is liquid – add more

flour.

• Make the burgers and place them together with the olive oil in the instant pot. • Set Manual mode (High pressure) for 1 minute (quick pressure release).

• It is recommended to serve burgers warm.

Nutrition:

• Calories 122, Fat 1.1, Fiber 8.7, Carbs 20.7, Protein 7.7

Scrumptious Baked Potatoes

• Preparation Time: 15-30 minutes | Cooking Time: 8 hours and 10 minutes | Servings: 8

Ingredients:

- 8 potatoes
- Salt to taste for serving
- Ground black pepper to taste for serving

Directions:

• Rinse potatoes until clean, wipe dry and then prick with a fork.

• Wrap each potato in an aluminum foil and place in a 6 to 8 quarts slow cooker. • Cover with a lid, and then plug in the slow cooker and let cook on a low heat setting for 8

hours or until tender.

• When the cooking time is over, unwrap potatoes and prick with a fork to check if potatoes

are tender or not.

• Sprinkle potatoes with salt, black pepper, and your favorite seasoning and serve.

Nutrition:

• Calories:93 Cal, Carbohydrates:3g, Protein:3g, Fats:1g, Fiber:2g.

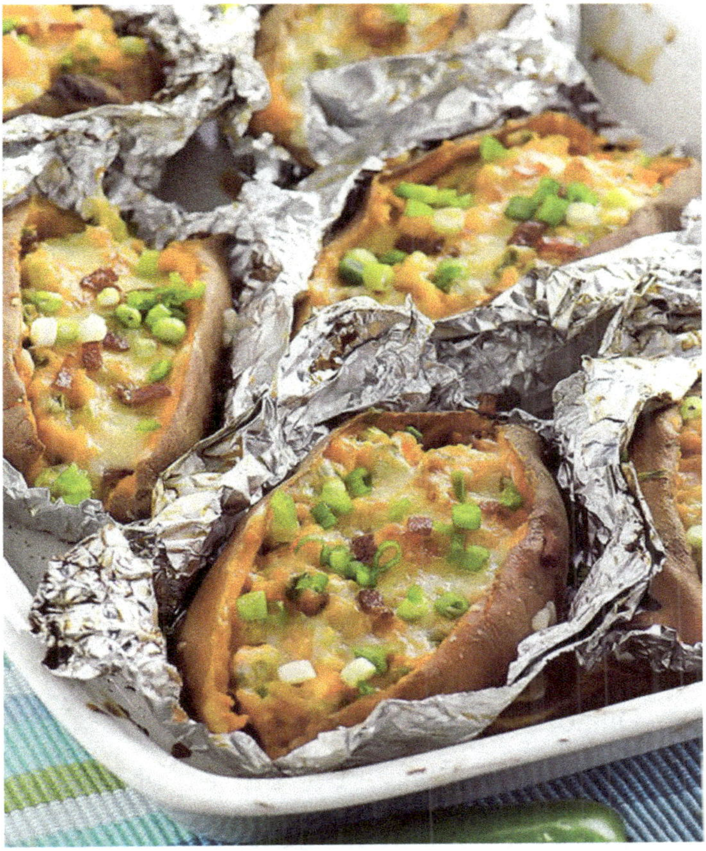

Fantastic Butternut Squash & Vegetables

• Preparation Time: 15-30 minutes | Cooking Time: 4 hours and 15 minutes | Servings: 6

Ingredients:

- 1 1/2 cups of corn kernels
- 2 pounds of butternut squash
- 1 medium-sized green bell pepper
- 14 1/2 ounce of diced tomatoes
- 1/2 cup of chopped white onion
- 1/2 teaspoon of minced garlic
- 1/2 teaspoon of salt
- 1/4 teaspoon of ground black pepper
- 1 tablespoon and 2 teaspoons of tomato paste
- 1/2 cup of vegetable broth

Directions:

• Peel, centralize the butternut squash and dice and place it into a 6-quarts slow cooker. • Create a hole on the green bell pepper, then cut it into 1/2 inch pieces and add it to the slow

cooker.

- Add the remaining ingredients into the slow cooker except for tomato paste, stir properly and cover it with the lid.
- Then plug in the slow cooker and let it cook on the low heat setting for 6 hours or until the vegetables get soft.
- When 6 hours of the cooking time is done, remove 1/2 cup of the cooking liquid from the slow cooker.
- Then pour the tomato mixture into this cooking liquid, stir properly and place it in the slow cooker.
- Stir properly and continue cooking for 30 minutes or until the mixture becomes slightly thick.
- Serve right away.

Nutrition:

- Calories:134 Cal, Carbohydrates:23g, Protein:6g, Fats:2g, Fiber:4g.

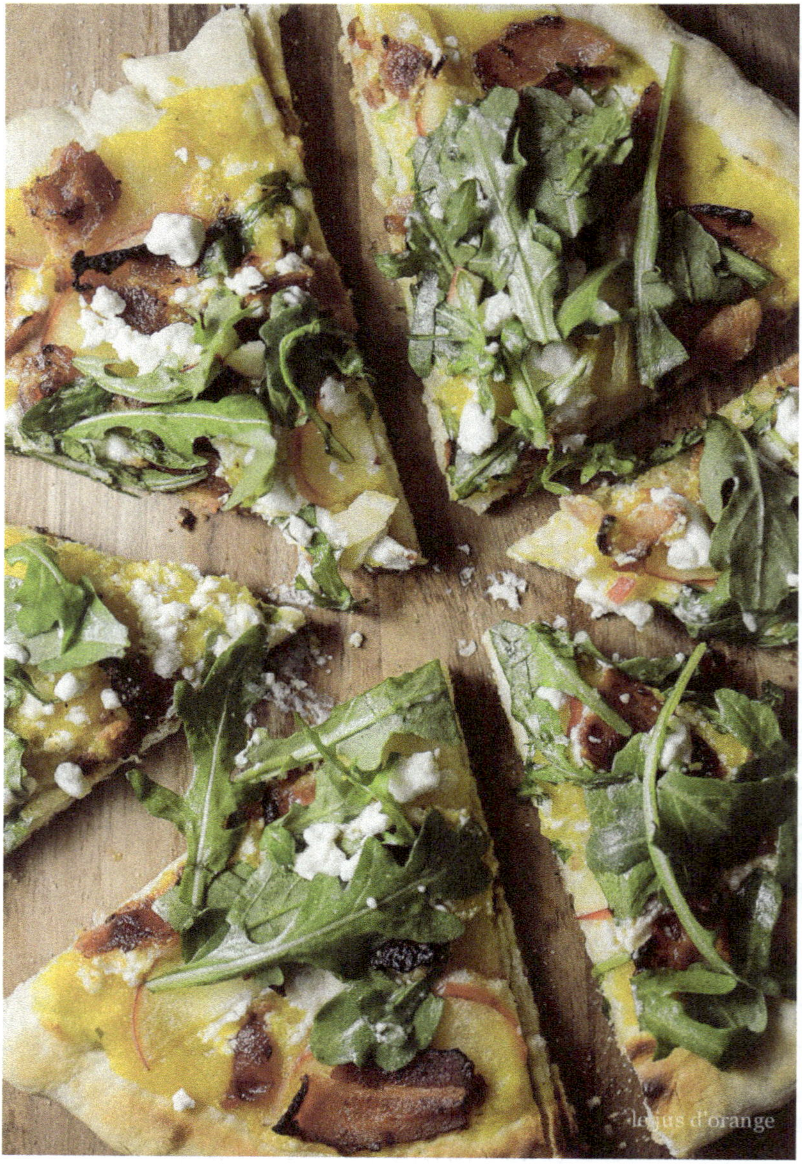
le jus d'orange

Balls from Beetroot

Preparation Time: 35 minutes | Cooking Time: 0 minutes | Servings: 4

Ingredients:

- 4 sprigs of parsley
- 2 tablespoon walnuts
- 260 g beetroot
- ½ onion
- 1 clove of garlic
- Salt and pepper

Directions:

- Boil the beetroot, peel, and grate coarsely with a kitchen grater.
- Roast the walnuts and process them into flour in a food processor.
- Cut the onion into small cubes, peel the garlic clove and mash it with a fork. • Wash, shake, and chop the parsley.

Mix all Ingredients: in a bowl and season with salt and a little pepper.

- Shape into balls of the same size and let stand

for a few minutes.

Nutrition:

- Calories: 239 Fat: 11.4g Carbs: 10.5g Protein: 12.1g Fiber: 3.2g

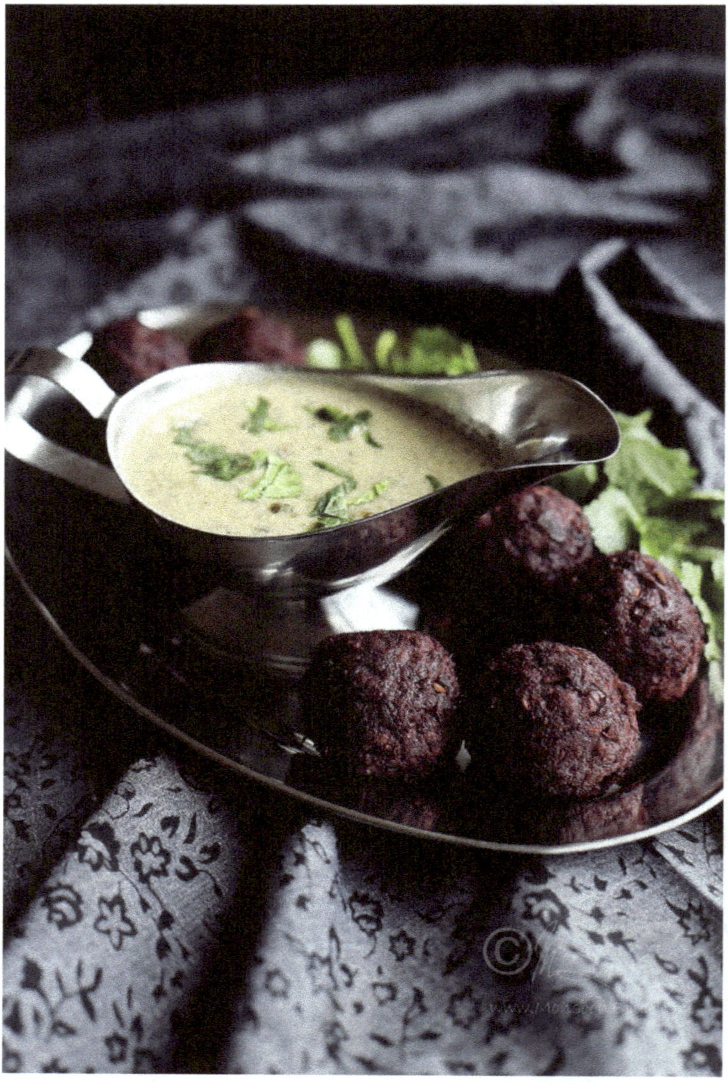

Polenta Skewers

Preparation Time: 35 minutes | Cooking Time: 0 minutes | Servings: 4

Ingredients:

- ½ avocado
- 10 cherry tomatoes
- 1 mini zucchini
- 150 g corn grits
- 2 tablespoon olive oil
- 1 teaspoon sesame seeds, black
- 10 basil leaves
- 10 toothpicks
- 450 ml of vegetable stock
- Salt and pepper

Directions:

- The day before, bring the corn grits to the boil in the broth and cook for a few minutes, stirring constantly. Pour into a square form and chill until the next day.
- Cut the polenta into small cubes and fry in a pan in a little olive oil.
- Wash the zucchini, cut into thin slices, and fry in

the pan once the polenta is ready.

- Wash the tomatoes and cut them in half, pluck the basil leaves from the branches.
- Stone the avocado and cut it into thin slices.
- Skewer a polenta cube, a zucchini, a tomato, a slice of avocado, and a basil leaf onto a toothpick. Serve with sesame seeds.

Nutrition:

- Calories: 259 Fat: 15.4g Carbs: 20.5g Protein: 12.1g Fiber: 3.2g

Börek with Spinach Filling

• Preparation Time: 25 minutes | Cooking Time: 0 minutes | Servings: 10

Ingredients:

- 10 yufka sheets
- 2 cloves of garlic
- 1 small onion
- 3 tablespoon soy yogurt
- 4 tablespoon soy milk
- 400 g spin nat
- 3 tablespoons of oil
- 1 pinch of nutmeg
- Salt and pepper

Directions:

- Wash the spinach, peel the garlic and onion and cut into small cubes.
- Steam the spinach, onion, and garlic in oil in a deep pan.
- After a few minutes, season with nutmeg, salt, and pepper and stir in the yogurt. • Lay the Yufka leaves and brush with the spinach filling.
- Roll up and brush with a little milk.

- Then place on a baking sheet and bake in the oven at 180 degrees Celsius for about 15

minutes.

Nutrition:

- Calories: 219 Fat: 9.4g Carbs: 10.5g Protein: 11.1g Fiber: 3.2g

Taler With Avocado Cream

Preparation Time: 25 minutes | Cooking Time: 0 minutes | Servings: 5

Ingredients:

- 20 pumpernickels, round
- 1 chili pepper
- 1 lime
- 2 avocados
- 6 beetroot chips
- 50 g vegan cream cheese
- Salt and pepper

Directions:

- Cut the chili pepper lengthways and scrape out the stones.
- Halve the avocados, core them and scrape the pulp into a blender jar.
- Add the cream cheese and a little lime juice.
- Mix a homogeneous cream from the chili pepper, avocado, lime, cream cheese, and a little

salt and pepper.

- Put the little Pumpernickel Taler ready and put a serving of avocado cream on each with a piping bag.
- Crumble the chips and sprinkle them over the talers.

Nutrition:

- Calories: 243 Fat: 10.4g Carbs: 12.5g Protein: 9.1g Fiber: 3.2g

Pumpernickel with Avocado

• Preparation Time: 10 minutes | Cooking Time: 0 minutes | Servings: 2

Ingredients:

- 6 small slices of pumpernickel
- 1 avocado
- 1 roll of vegan cheese spread
- 1 tablespoon chives
- Salt and pepper

Directions:

- Halve the avocado, remove the seeds, and carefully remove them from the skin. Cut into slices and place on a plate.
- Spread cheese on the bread, then top with avocado, and then sprinkle with a little pepper and chopped chives.

Nutrition:

- Calories: 159 Fat: 9.4g Carbs: 10.5g Protein: 9.1g Fiber: 3.2g

Savory Mushroom Cakes

Preparation Time: 30 minutes | Cooking Time: 0 minutes | Servings: 4

Ingredients:

- 1 bun
- 1 small onion
- 1 clove of garlic
- 500 g mushrooms
- 1 pinch of marjoram
- 2 tablespoons of oil
- 1 tablespoon flaxseed, crushed
- 3 tablespoon soy milk
- Salt and pepper

Directions:

- Clean the mushrooms and cut them into small cubes. Peel the onion and garlic, then also dice.
- Crumble the bun and mix in a bowl with the mushrooms, garlic, and onion.
- Add marjoram, salt, and pepper, and fold in the flax seeds as well.
- Add soy milk so that the mixture sticks well.
- Heat the oil in a non-stick pan, form small

meatballs and fry them until golden brown on both sides.

Nutrition:

- Calories: 129 Fat: 12.4g Carbs: 11.5g Protein: 9.1g Fiber: 3.2g

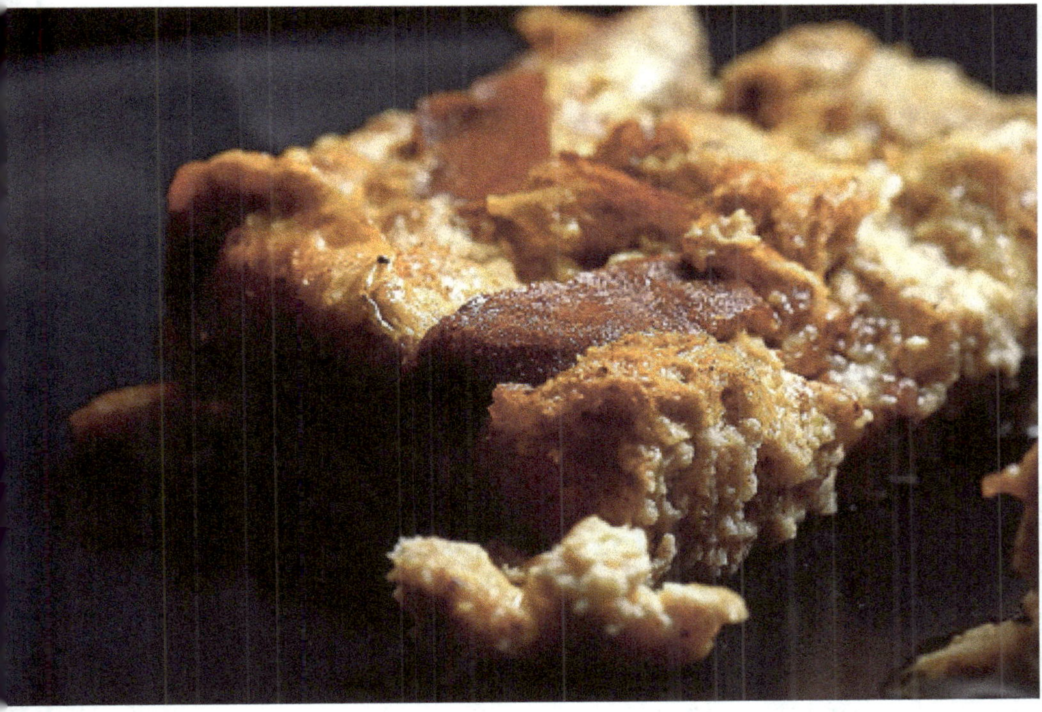

Churros With Chocolate

Preparation Time: 35 minutes | Cooking Time: 0 minutes | Servings: 6

Ingredients:

- 2 teaspoons of baking powder
- 1 ¼ cup of flour
- 2 cups of oil
- 1 pinch of salt
- 50 g sugar
- 1 cup of soy milk
- 100 g vegan chocolate
- cinnamon and sugar

Directions:

- Mix the sugar, baking powder, flour, and salt. Then stir in ¾ of the soy milk until a velvety batter is formed.
- Heat the oil in a saucepan and roll the churro batter into a long line.
- When the oil is hot, cut the thin roll into pieces with scissors and bake them in the oil until they are evenly golden yellow on all sides.

- In Zimt and roll sugar and heat the chocolate with the remaining soy milk.

Nutrition:

- Calories: 209 Fat: 15.4g Carbs: 20.5g Protein: 12.1g Fiber: 3.2g

Zucchini Rolls with Cream Cheese

Preparation Time: 35 minutes | Cooking Time: 0 minutes | Servings: 4

Ingredients:

- 1 tablespoon oil
- 60 g apricots, dried
- 350 g zucchini
- Salt and pepper
- 1 sprig of thyme
- ½ lime

Directions:

- Turn after a minute and fry the same way on the other side.
- Let cool on a plate and in the meantime prepare the filling.
- Let the apricots soak a little and then chop them.
- Mix with cream cheese, chopped thyme, and a little pepper. Season to taste with salt and

prepare.

- Brush the zucchini slices with some filling and roll-up.
- Add a few squirts of lime juice to serve.

Nutrition:

- Calories: 235 Fat: 15.4g Carbs: 20.5g Protein: 12.1g Fiber: 3.2g

Spinach Burgers

• Preparation Time: 10 minutes | Cooking Time: 10 minutes | Servings: 7

Ingredients:

- 3 cups spinach, chopped
- 2 tablespoon coconut shreds
- 4 tablespoon panko breadcrumbs
- 1 teaspoon salt
- 1/2 teaspoon chili flakes
- 2 tablespoon flax meal
- 6 tablespoon hot water
- 1 teaspoon olive oil
- 1 tablespoon coconut yogurt

Directions:

• In the mixing bowl mix up together flax meal and hot water. Whisk the mixture. • Then add coconut shred, panko breadcrumbs, spinach, chili flakes, coconut yogurt, and salt. • Mix up the mixture until homogenous.

• Set the Saute mode in Instant pot and preheat it until it shows —Hot‖.

• Then brush the instant bowl with olive oil from

inside.

- Make patties from the spinach mixture with the help of 2 spoons and place them in the

instant pot.

- Saute them for 10 minutes. You can flip the patties during cooking if desired. Nutrition:
- Calories: 47, Fat: 2.9, Fiber: 1.3, Carbs: 4.5, Protein: 1.5

Tempeh Patties

• Preparation Time: 15 minutes | Cooking Time: 11 minutes | Servings: 5

Ingredients:

- 10 oz tempeh
- 1 carrot, peeled
- 4 tablespoon oatmeal
- 1/4 teaspoon minced garlic
- 1 teaspoon onion powder
- 1/2 teaspoon salt
- 2 oz black beans, canned
- 1 tablespoon tomato sauce
- 1 teaspoon golden syrup
- 1/2 cup water, for cooking

Directions:

- Cut tempeh into chunks and place it on the steamer rack.
- Pour water into the instant pot and insert the steamer rack with tempeh.
- Close the lid and cook on Manual mode (High pressure) for 7 minutes. Then use quick

pressure release.

- Meanwhile, chop the carrot and place it in the food processor.
- Add minced garlic, oatmeal onion powder, salt, canned beans, tomato sauce, and golden

syrup.

- Blend the mixture for 2-3 minutes.
- Then add cooked tempeh and keep blending for 1 minute more. The final mixture texture

shouldn't be too smooth.

- Use the burger mold and make burgers. Freeze them until solid.
- Then wrap every burger in foil or use non-stick paper and place in the cleaned instant pot

bowl.

- Cook the burgers on High (Manual mode) for 4 minutes. Then allow natural pressure release for 10 minutes.

Nutrition:

• Calories: 175, Fat: 6.6, Fiber: 2.5, Carbs: 18, Protein: 13.7

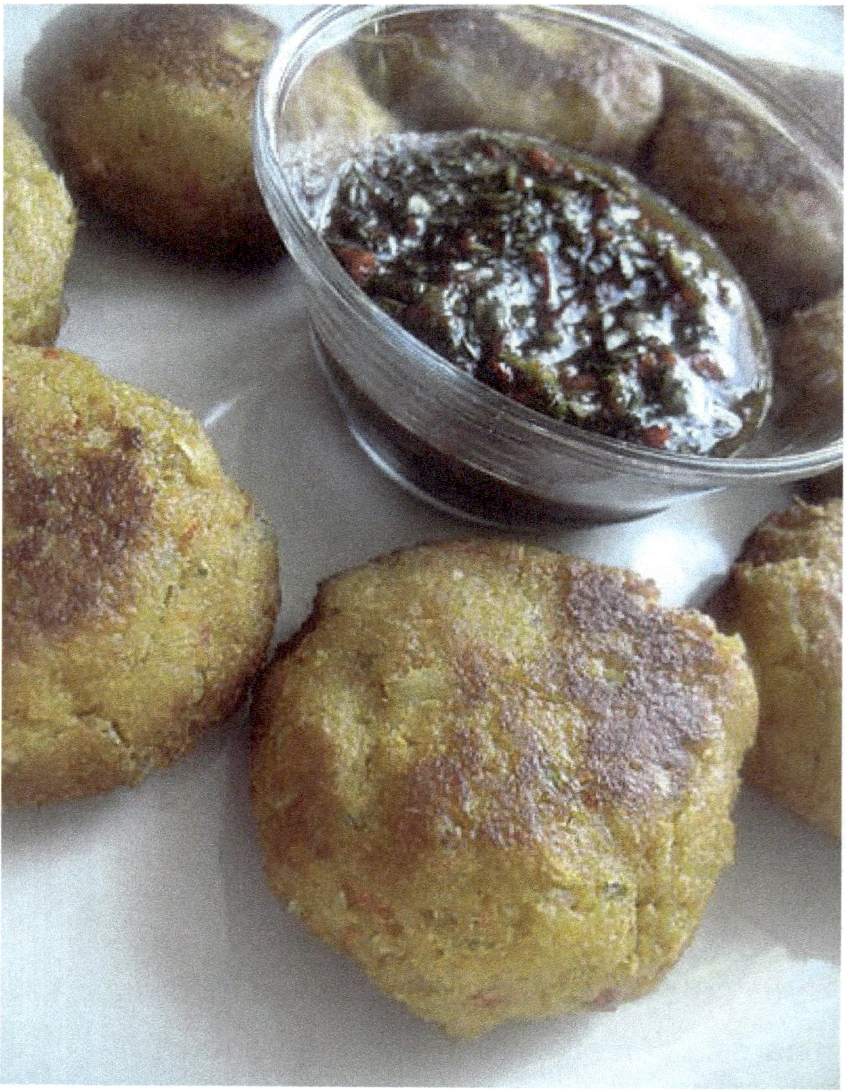

Pumpkin Burgers

Preparation Time: 10 minutes | Cooking Time: 3 minutes | Servings: 2

Ingredients:

- 2 hamburger buns
- 1 tablespoon pumpkin seeds
- 1 tablespoon pumpkin powder
- 3 tablespoon pumpkin puree
- 2 tablespoons breadcrumbs
- 1/2 teaspoon chili flakes
- 1 teaspoon turmeric
- 1 tablespoon flax meal
- 3 tablespoons hot water

Directions:

- In the mixing bowl combine flax meal and hot water. Whisk the mixture and add pumpkin powder, pumpkin puree, breadcrumbs, chili flakes, and turmeric.
- Mix up the mixture. Add pumpkin seeds.
- With the help of the burger mold, make 2 burgers.
- Place them in the instant pot bowl and close the

lid.

- Set Manual mode (High pressure) and cook for 3 minutes.
- Then use quick pressure release and open the lid.
- Fill the burger buns with pumpkin burgers.

Nutrition:

- Calories: 197, Fat: 5.6, Fiber: 3.3, Carbs: 30.5, Protein: 7.2

Fabulous Glazed Carrots

• Preparation Time: 15-30 minutes | Cooking Time: 2 hours and 20 minutes | Servings: 5

Ingredients:

- 1 pound of carrots
- 2 teaspoons of chopped cilantro
- 1/4 teaspoon of salt
- 1/4 cup of brown sugar
- 1/4 teaspoon of ground cinnamon
- 1/8 teaspoon of ground nutmeg
- 1 tablespoon of cornstarch
- 1 tablespoon of olive oil
- 2 tablespoons of water
- 1 large orange, juiced and zested

Directions:

- Peel the carrots, rinse, cut them into 1/4 inch thick rounds and place them in a 6 quarts slow cooker.
- Add the salt, sugar, cinnamon, nutmeg, olive oil, orange zest, juice, and stir properly.
- Cover it with the lid, then plug in the slow cooker and let it cook on the high heat setting for 2 hours

or until the carrots become soft.

- Stir properly the cornstarch and water until it blends well. Thereafter, add this mixture to the slow cooker.
- Continue cooking for 10 minutes or until the sauce in the slow cooker gets slightly thick.
- Sprinkle the cilantro over carrots and serve.

Nutrition:

- Calories:160 Cal, Carbohydrates:40g, Protein:1g, Fats:0. 3g, Fiber:2. 3g.

Flavorful Sweet Potatoes with Apples

• Preparation Time: 15-30 minutes | Cooking Time: 5 hours | Servings: 6

Ingredients:

- 3 medium-sized apples, peeled and cored
- 6 medium-sized sweet potatoes, peeled and cored
- 1/4 cup of pecans
- 1/4 teaspoon of ground cinnamon
- 1/4 teaspoon of ground nutmeg
- 2 tablespoons of vegan butter, melted
- 1/4 cup of maple syrup

Directions:

- Cut the sweet potatoes and the apples into 1/2 inch slices.
- Grease a 6-quarts slow cooker with a non-stick cooking spray and arrange the sweet potato

slices in the bottom of the cooker.

- Top it with the apple slices; sprinkle it with the cinnamon and nutmeg, before garnishing it with butter.
- Cover it with the lid, plug in the slow cooker and let it cook on the low heat setting for 4 hours or until the sweet potatoes get soft.
- When done, sprinkle it with pecans and continue cooking for another 30 minutes. • Serve right away.

Nutrition:

- Calories:120 Cal, Carbohydrates:24g, Protein:1g, Fats:3g, Fiber:2g.

Buttery Baby Potatoes

• Preparation Time: 15-30 minutes | Cooking Time: 40 minutes | Servings: 4

Ingredients:

- 4 tbsp unsalted plant butter, melted
- 4 garlic cloves, minced
- 3 tbsp chopped chives
- Salt and black pepper to taste
- 2 tbsp grated plant-based Parmesan cheese
- 1 ½ lb baby potatoes, rinsed and drained

Directions:

- Preheat the oven to 400 F.
- In a large bowl, mix the butter, garlic, chives, salt, black pepper, and plant Parmesan cheese.

Toss the potatoes in the butter mixture until well coated.

- Spread the mixture into a baking sheet, cover with foil, and roast in the oven for 30 minutes or until tender.

- Remove the potatoes from the oven and toss in the remaining butter mixture. Serve.

Nutrition:

- Calories 192 kcal Fats 8. 8g Carbs 25. 7g Protein 4. 1g

Sweetened Carrots With Parsley Drizzle

• Preparation Time: 15-30 minutes | Cooking Time: 14 minutes | Servings: 4

Ingredients:

- 1 lb baby carrots
- 2 tbsp plant butter
- 2 tbsp pure maple syrup
- 1 tbsp freshly squeezed lemon juice
- ½ tsp black pepper
- ¼ cup chopped fresh parsley

Directions:

- Boil some water in a medium pot. Add some salt and cook the carrots until tender, 5 to 6 minutes. Drain the carrots.
- Melt the butter in a large skillet and mix in the maple syrup and lemon juice.
- Toss in the carrots, season with black pepper, and toss in the parsley.
- Serve the carrots.

Nutrition:

- Calories 120 kcal Fats 6g Carbs 16. 8g Protein 1. 1g

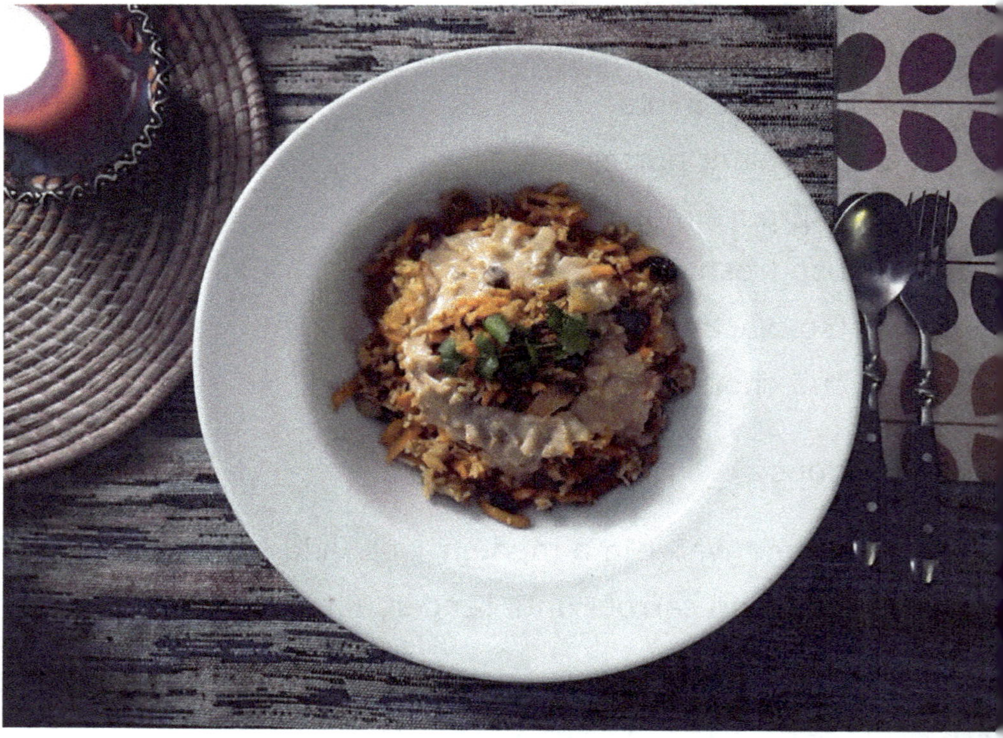

Chipotle and Lime Tortilla Chips

• Preparation Time: 10 minutes | Cooking Time: 15 minutes | Servings: 4

Ingredients:

- 12 ounces whole-wheat tortillas
- 4 tablespoons chipotle seasoning 1 tablespoon olive oil
- 4 limes, juiced

Directions:

- Whisk together oil and lime juice, brush it well on tortillas, then sprinkle with chipotle seasoning and bake for 15 minutes at 350 degrees F until crispy, turning halfway.
- When done, let the tortilla cool for 10 minutes, then break it into chips and serve.

Nutrition:

- Calories: 150 Cal Fat: 7 g Carbs: 18 g Protein: 2 g Fiber: 2 g

Carrot and Sweet Potato Fritters

• Preparation Time: 10 minutes | Cooking Time: 8 minutes | Servings: 10

Ingredients:

- 1/3 cup quinoa flour
- 1½ cups shredded sweet potato
- 1 cup grated carrot
- 1/3 teaspoon ground black pepper
- 2/3 teaspoon salt
- 2 teaspoons curry powder
- 2 flax eggs
- 2 tablespoons coconut oil

Directions:

- Place all the ingredients in a bowl, except for oil, stir well until combined, and then shape the mixture into ten small patties
- Take a large pan, place it over medium-high heat, add oil and when it melts, add patties in it and cook for 3 minutes per side until browned.
- Serve straight away

Nutrition:

- Calories: 70 Cal Fat: 3 g Carbs: 8 g Protein: 1 g

Fiber: 1 g

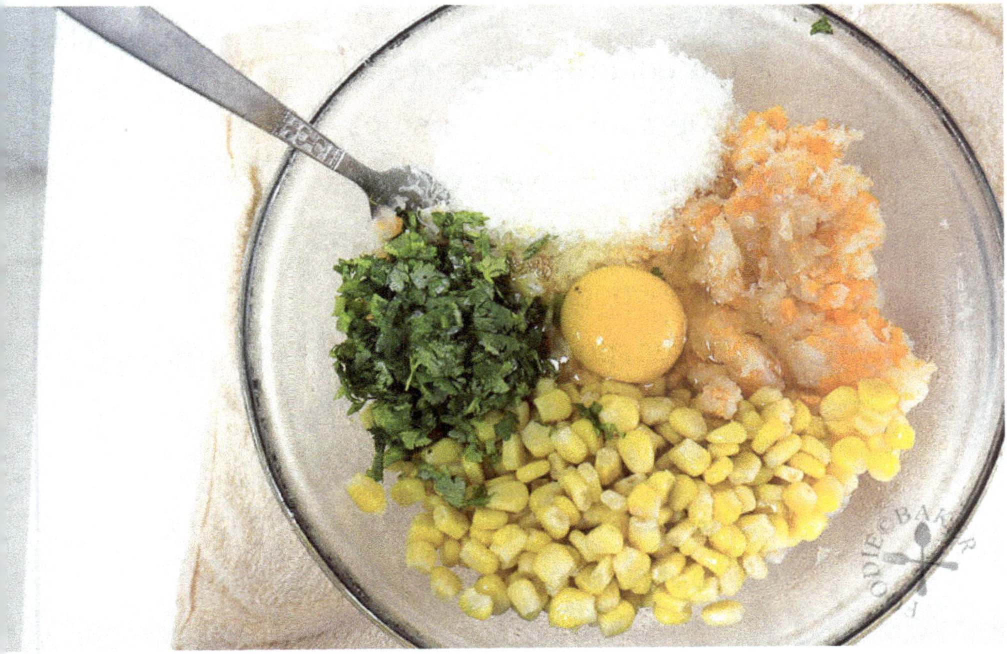

Wonderful Glazed Root Vegetables

• Preparation Time: 15-30 minutes | Cooking Time: 4 hours and 20 minutes | Servings: 6

Ingredients:

- 6 medium-sized carrots
- 4 medium-sized parsnips
- 1 pound of sweet potatoes
- 2 medium-sized red onions
- 1 teaspoon of salt
- 1/2 teaspoon of ground black pepper
- 5 teaspoons of chopped thyme
- 3 tablespoons of honey
- 1 tablespoon of apple cider vinegar
- 1 tablespoon of olive oil

Directions:

• Peel the carrots, parsnip, sweet potatoes, onions, and cut them into 1-inch pieces. • Grease a 6 quarts slow cooker with a non-stick cooking spray, place the carrots, parsnip, onion in the bottom and then top it with the sweet potatoes.

• Using a bowl whisk the salt, black pepper, 2 teaspoons of thyme, honey, and oil properly. • Pour this mixture over on the vegetables and toss it to coat.

• Cover it with the lid, then plug in the slow cooker and let it cook at the low heat setting for 4

hours or until the vegetables get tender.

• When cooked, pour in the vinegar, stir, sprinkle it with the remaining thyme and serve. Nutrition:

• Calories:137 Cal, Carbohydrates:26g, Protein:2g, Fats:4g, Fiber:3g.

Super Aubergines

• Preparation Time: 15-30 minutes | Cooking Time: 8 hours and 15 minutes | Servings: 6

Ingredients:

- 1 pound of eggplant
- 10-ounce of tomatoes, quartered
- 2-ounce of sun-dried tomatoes
- 1 small fennel bulb, sliced
- 1 medium-sized red onion, peeled and sliced
- 1/2 cup of chopped parsley
- 1/4 cup of chopped basil
- 1/4 cup of chopped chives
- 2 teaspoons of capers
- 1 teaspoon of minced garlic
- 1 1/2 teaspoon of salt
- 1 teaspoon of ground black pepper
- 1 teaspoon of coriander seeds
- 1 lemon, juiced
- 6 tablespoons of olive oil, divided

Directions:

- Using a 6 quarts slow cooker, add 2

tablespoons of olive oil, top it with onions and garlic. • Remove the stem of the eggplant, cut it into 1/2-inch thick slices and brush 2 tablespoons of

oil on both sides of the eggplant slices.

- Garnish the onion with the eggplant slices and cover it with tomato pieces, sun-dried tomatoes, and fennel slices.
- Sprinkle it with salt, black pepper, and coriander seeds.
- Cover it with the lid, then plug in the slow cooker and let it cook at the low heat setting for 6 to 8 hours or until vegetables get tender.
- While doing that, place the parsley, basil, and chives in a food processor.
- Add the remaining 2 tablespoons of olive oil along with the lemon juice, caper, and pulse it until it gets smooth.
- When the vegetables are cooked, transfer them to a serving platter and drizzle them with the prepared herbs mixture.
- Serve right away with crusty bread.

Nutrition:

- Calories:62 Cal, Carbohydrates:12g, Protein:2g, Fats:2g, Fiber:4g.

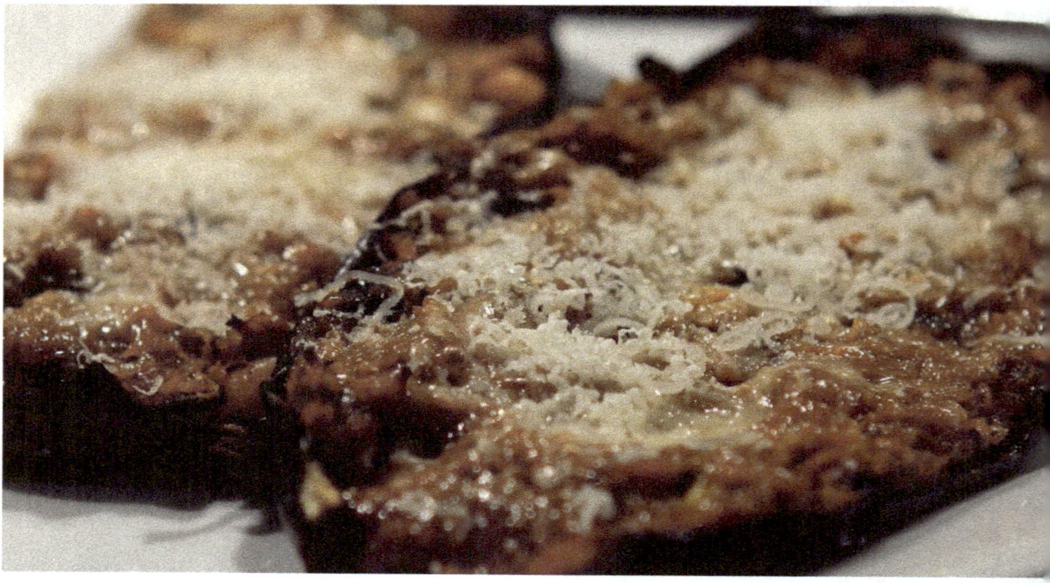

Sweet and Spicy Red Thai Vegetable Curry

• Preparation Time: 15-30 minutes | Cooking Time: 4 hours and 45 minutes | Servings: 6

Ingredients:

- 1/2 head cauliflower, chopped into florets
- 2 medium-sized sweet potatoes, peeled and cubed
- 1 cup of cooked green peas
- 8 ounce of chopped white mushrooms
- 1/4 cup of chopped cilantro, chopped
- 1 small white onion, sliced
- 1/2 teaspoon of salt
- 1 tablespoon of brown sugar
- 1/2 cup of toasted cashews
- 3 tablespoon of red curry paste
- 3 tablespoons of soy sauce
- 2 teaspoons of Sriracha sauce
- 14-ounce of coconut milk

Directions:

- Grease a 6-quarts slow cooker with a non-stick cooking spray and add the cauliflower florets, sweet potatoes, and onion.
- Using a bowl, stir properly the salt, sugar, red curry paste, soy sauce, Sriracha sauce, and coconut milk.
- Pour this mixture on top of the vegetables in the slow cooker and toss it to coat properly.
- Cover it with the lid, then plug in the slow cooker and let it cook at the low heat setting for 4 hours or until the vegetables get soft.
- Then add the mushrooms, peas, to the slow cooker and continue cooking for 30 minutes.
- Garnish it with cilantro and serve.

Nutrition:

- Calories:141 Cal, Carbohydrates:13g, Protein:0g, Fats:9g, Fiber:3g.

Vibrant Minestrone

• Preparation Time: 15-30 minutes | Cooking Time: 6 hours and 25 minutes | Servings: 6

Ingredients:

- 30 ounce of cooked cannellini beans
- 8 ounces of uncooked small pasta
- 12 thin asparagus spears
- 3 carrots, peeled and sliced
- 6 ounce of chopped spinach
- 28 ounce of diced tomatoes
- 1 cup of cooked peas
- 1 medium-sized white onion, peeled and diced
- 1 1/2 teaspoon of minced garlic
- 1 teaspoon of salt
- 1/2 teaspoon of ground black pepper
- 3 cups of vegetable stock
- 3 cups of water
- 1/3 cup of grated parmesan cheese

Directions:

• Grease a 6-quarts slow cooker with a non-stick cooking spray, add the beans, carrots, tomatoes, onion, garlic, vegetable stock, and water.

- Stir properly and cover it with the lid.
- Then plug in the slow cooker and let it cook at the low heat setting for 4 hours or until the vegetables get soft.
- While doing that cut the asparagus into three and when the vegetables are cooked add the asparagus to the slow cooker along with the peas, salt, black pepper, spinach, and pasta.
- Continue cooking for 15 minutes.
- Garnish it with cheese and serve.

Nutrition:

- Calories:110 Cal, Carbohydrates:18g, Protein:5g, Fats:2g, Fiber:4g.

Broccoli Tots

• Preparation Time: 15-30 minutes | Cooking Time: 30 minutes | Servings: 4

Ingredients:

- 1 tbsp flax seed powder + 3 tbsp water
- 1 large head broccoli, cut into florets
- 2/3 cup toasted almond flour
- 2 garlic cloves, minced
- 2 cups grated plant-based Parmesan cheese
- Salt to taste

Directions:

- Preheat the oven to 350 F and line a baking sheet with parchment paper.
- In a small bowl, mix the flax seed powder with the water and allow thickening for 5 minutes to make the flax egg.
- Place the broccoli in a safe microwave bowl, sprinkle with 2 tbsp of water, and steam in the microwave for 1 minute or until softened.

• Transfer the broccoli to a food processor and add the flax egg, almond flour, garlic, plant cheese, and salt. Blend until coarsely smooth and well combined.

• Pour the mixture into a bowl and form 2-inch oblong balls from the mixture. • Place the tots on the baking sheet and bake in the oven for 15 to 20 minutes or until firm and compacted.

• Remove the tots from the oven and serve warm with tomato dipping sauce.

Nutrition:

• Calories 216 Fats 14. 08g Carbs 7. 78g Protein 14. 66g

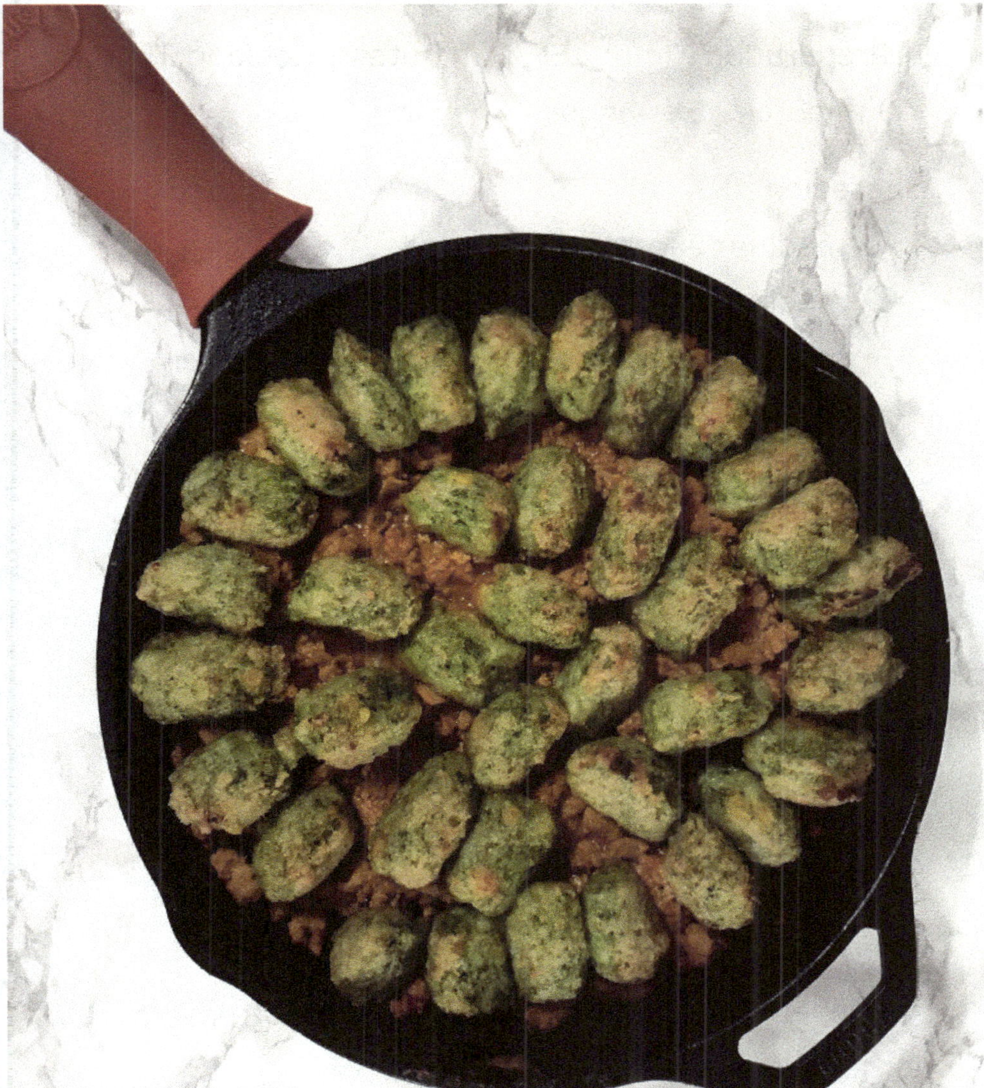

Summer Vegetable Mix

• Preparation Time: 15-30 minutes | Cooking Time: 40 minutes | Servings: 4

Ingredients:

- 2 medium zucchinis, chopped
- 2 medium yellow squash, chopped
- 1 medium red onion, cut into 1-inch wedges
- 1 medium red bell pepper, deseeded and cut into 1-inch dices
- 1 cup cherry tomatoes, halved
- 4 tbsp olive oil
- Salt and black pepper to taste
- 3 garlic cloves, minced
- 2/3 cup whole-wheat breadcrumbs
- 1 lemon, zested
- ¼ cup chopped fresh basil

Directions:

- Preheat the oven to 450 F and lightly grease a large baking sheet with cooking spray.

- In a medium bowl, add the zucchini, yellow squash, red onion, bell pepper, tomatoes, olive oil, salt, black pepper, and garlic. Toss well and spread the mixture on the baking sheet.

- Roast in the oven for 25 to 30 minutes or until the vegetables are tender while stirring every 5 minutes.
- Meanwhile, heat the olive oil in a medium skillet and sauté the garlic until fragrant. Mix in the breadcrumbs, lemon zest, and basil. Cook for 2 to 3 minutes.
- Remove the vegetables from the oven and toss in the breadcrumb's mixture.
- Serve warm.

Nutrition:

- Calories 258 kcal Fats 14. 5g Carbs 30. 4g Protein 5. 5g

Mixed Seed Crackers

• Preparation Time: 15-30 minutes | Cooking Time: 50 minutes | Servings: 4

Ingredients:

- 1/3 cup coconut flour
- 1/3 cup sesame seeds
- 1/3 cup sunflower seeds
- 1/3 cup chia seeds
- 1/3 cup pumpkin seeds
- 1 tsp salt
- ¼ cup plant butter, melted
- 1 cup boiling water

Directions:

- Preheat an oven to 300 F and line a baking sheet with parchment paper.
- In a medium bowl, mix the coconut flour, sesame seeds, sunflower seeds, chia seeds, pumpkin seeds, and salt.
- Add the plant butter, boiling water, and mix until well combined.
- Spread the mixture on the baking sheet

and bake in the oven for 45 minutes until the crackers

are firm.

- Remove the crackers and allow cooling for 10 minutes.
- Break the crackers into pieces and enjoy!

Nutrition:

- Calories 725 Fats 67. 2g Carbs 18. 1g Protein 24. 3g

Seitan Bell Pepper Balls

• Preparation Time: 15-30 minutes | Cooking Time: 25 minutes | Servings: 4

Ingredients:

- 1 tbsp flax seed powder + 3 tbsp water
- 1 lb seitan, crumbled
- ¼ cup chopped mixed bell peppers
- Salt and black pepper to taste
- 1 tbsp almond flour
- 1 tsp garlic powder
- 1 tsp onion powder
- 1 tsp tofu mayonnaise
- Olive oil for brushing

Directions:

• Preheat the oven to 400 F and line a baking sheet with parchment paper.

• In a medium bowl, mix the flax seed powder with water and allow thickening for 5 minutes. • Add the seitan, bell peppers, salt, black pepper, almond flour, garlic powder, onion powder, and tofu mayonnaise. Mix well and form 1-inch balls from the mixture.

- Arrange on the baking sheet, brush with cooking spray, and bake in the oven for 15 to 20 minutes or until brown and compacted.
- Remove from the oven and serve.

Nutrition:

- Calories 492 Fats 41. 3g Carbs 4. 1g Protein 26. 5g

Quinoa Stuffed Tomatoes

• Preparation Time: 15-30 minutes | Cooking Time: 50 minutes | Servings: 4

Ingredients:

- 8 medium-sized tomatoes
- ¾ cup quinoa, rinsed and drained
- 1 ½ cups water
- 1 tbsp olive oil
- 1 small onion, diced
- 3 garlic cloves, minced
- Salt and black pepper to taste
- 1 cup chopped spinach
- 1 (7 oz) can chickpeas, drained and rinsed
- ½ cup chopped fresh basil

Directions:

- Preheat the oven to 400 F.
- Cut off the heads of tomatoes and use a paring knife to scoop the inner pulp of the tomatoes.

Season with some olive oil, salt, and black pepper.

- Add the quinoa and water to a medium pot, season with salt, and cook for 10 to 15 minutes until the quinoa is tender and the water is absorbed. Fluff and set aside.
- Heat the remaining olive oil in a medium skillet and sauté the onion and garlic until softened and fragrant, 30 seconds.
- Mix in the spinach and cook until wilted, 2 minutes. Stir in the basil, chickpeas, and quinoa; allow warming from 2 minutes.
- Spoon the mixture into the tomatoes, place the tomatoes into the baking dish and bake in the oven for 20 minutes or until the tomatoes soften. Remove the tomatoes from the oven and dish the food. Serve warm.

Nutrition:

- Calories 296 kcal Fats 7. 5g Carbs 48. 3g Protein 12g

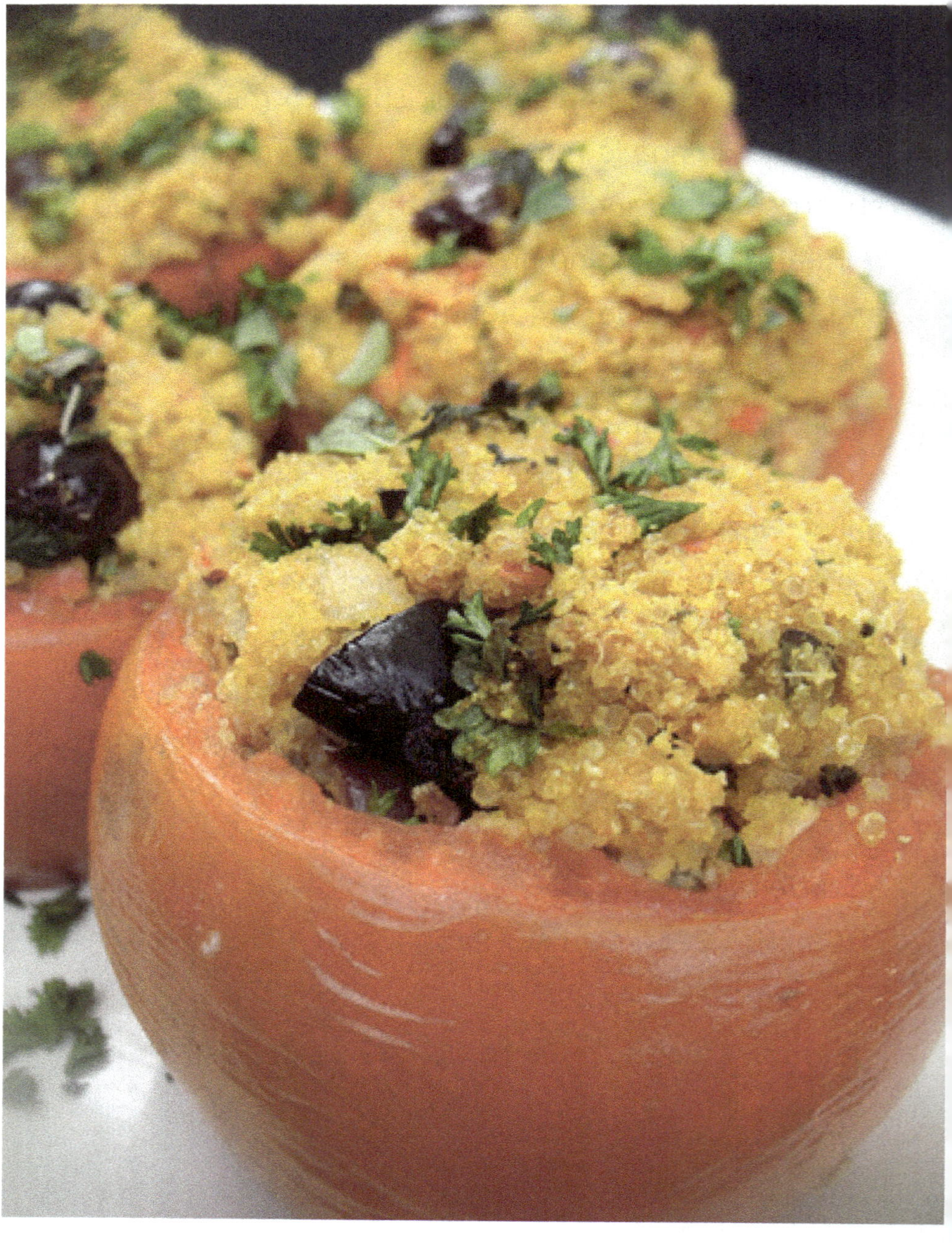

Cajun Sweet Potato Chips

• Preparation Time: 15-30 minutes | Cooking Time: 55 minutes | Servings: 4

Ingredients:

- 2 sweet potatoes, peeled and thinly sliced
- Salt to season
- 2 tbsp melted plant butter
- 1 tbsp Cajun seasoning

Directions:

- Preheat the oven to 400 F and line a baking sheet with parchment paper.
- In a medium bowl, add the sweet potatoes, salt, plant butter, and Cajun seasoning. Toss well.

Spread the chips on the baking sheet making sure not to overlap and bake in the oven for 50 minutes to 1 hour or until crispy.

- Remove the sheet and pour the chips into a large bowl.
- Allow cooling and enjoy.

Nutrition:

- Calories 65 Fats 5. 9g Carbs 2. 8g Protein 1g

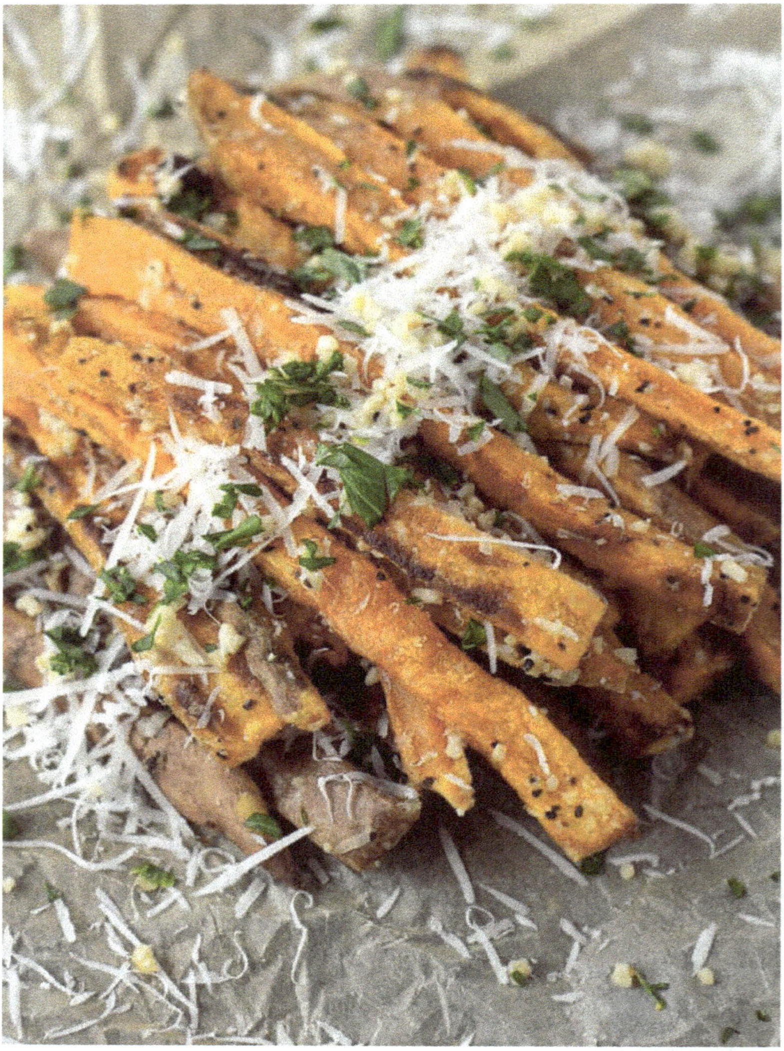

Maple Cinnamon Popcorn

• Preparation Time: 15-30 minutes | Cooking Time: 15 minutes | Servings: 4

Ingredients:

- ½ cup popcorn kernels
- ¼ tsp cinnamon powder
- ½ tsp pure maple syrup
- 1 tsp plant butter, melted
- Salt to taste

Directions:

• Pour the popcorn kernels into a large pot and set over medium heat. Cover the lid and allow the kernels to pop completely. Shake the pot a few times to ensure even popping, 10 minutes.

• Meanwhile, in a small bowl, mix the cinnamon powder, maple syrup, butter, and salt. When the popcorn is ready, turn the heat off, and toss in the cinnamon mixture until well distributed. Pour the popcorn into serving bowls, allow cooling, and enjoy.

Nutrition:

- Calories 15 Fats 1g Carbs 1. 5g Protein 0. 2g

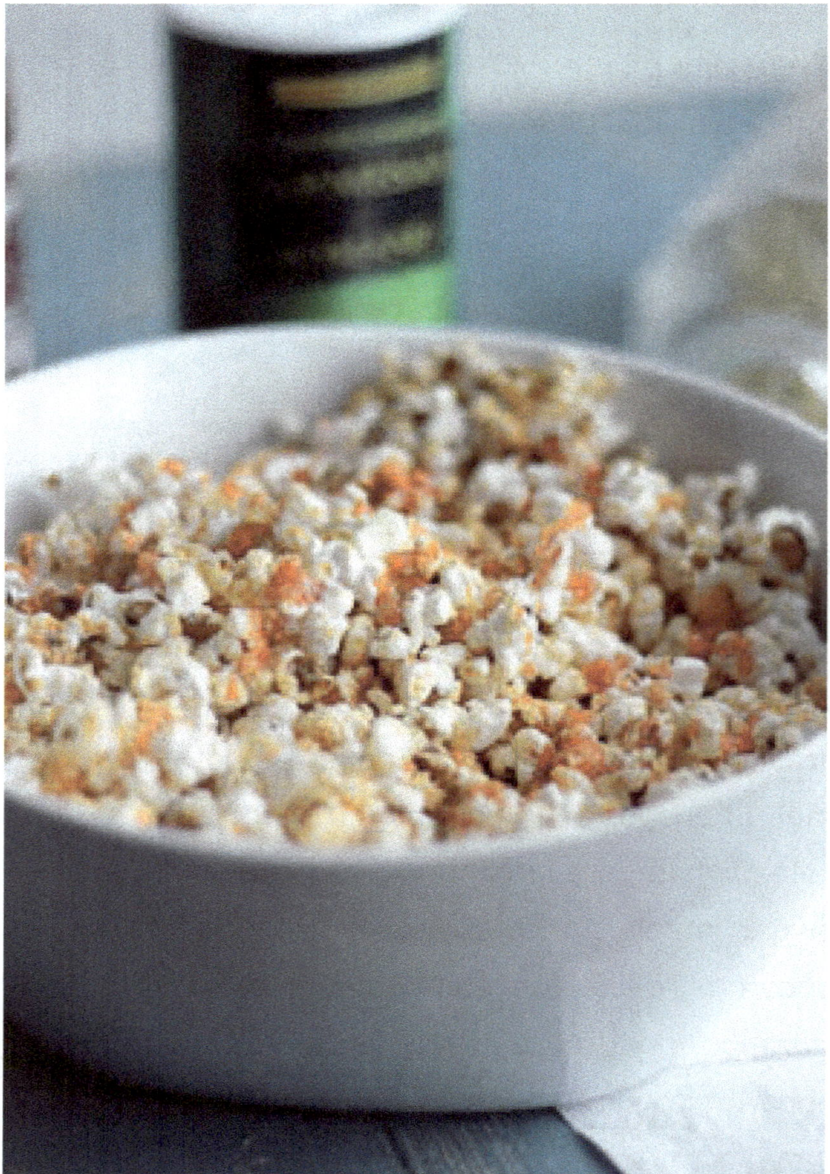

Skewers of Mozzarella And Tomato

• Preparation Time: 15 minutes | Cooking Time: 0 minutes | Servings: 8

- 1 teaspoon pesto
- 250 g cherry tomatoes
- 250 g vegan mozzarella
- 1 bunch of basil
- 3 tablespoon olive oil

Directions:

- Wash and prepare the tomatoes.
- Pluck the basil leaves, cut the mozzarella into small cubes.
- Mix the pesto with the olive oil in a small bowl.
- Prepare wooden skewers and place two tomatoes, two basil leaves, and two cubes of

mozzarella alternately on the skewers.

- Brush with a little pesto to serve.

Nutrition:

- Calories: 259 Fat: 15.4g Carbs: 20.5g Protein: 12.1g Fiber: 3.2g

Filled Mushrooms

Preparation Time: 55 minutes | Cooking Time: 0 minutes | Servings: 2

Ingredients:

- 30 g pine nuts
- ½ lime
- ½ bunch of basil
- 8 large mushrooms
- 50 ml of water
- 115 g cashew nuts
- 2 tablespoon coconut milk
- Salt and pepper

Directions:

- Soak the cashew nuts in water the evening before.
- The drain water and fill the cores together with the basil, the coconut milk, the water, and the lime juice in a food processor.
- Process into a creamy puree.
- Clean the mushrooms and brush with the filling.

- Then bake in the oven at 180 degrees Celsius for about 15 minutes.
- In the meantime, toast the pine nuts in a small non-stick pan.
- Sprinkle the pine nuts over the mushrooms to serve.

Nutrition:

- Calories: 239 Fat: 11.4g Carbs: 10.5g Protein: 11.1g Fiber: 3.2g

Pizza Bites

Preparation Time: 95 minutes | Cooking Time: 0 minutes | Servings: 8

- 200 g flour
- 1 teaspoon salt
- 180 ml of water
- ½ cubes of yeast
- 1 teaspoon of sugar
- 250 g vegan salami
- 250 g vegan Gouda

Directions:

- Mix sugar, flour, and salt in a bowl.
- Make a well and crumble the yeast into it. Warm the water slightly and gradually pour it into the hollow.
- Mix the yeast and let it rise briefly, then work all the Ingredients in the bowl into a smooth dough.
- Let rise for 50 minutes, then roll out.
- Cut the cheese and salami into thin slices.

- Cut rectangles from the dough and cover the lower edge with cheese and salami. Roll up a little, cover again, and close the dough.
- Bake at 240 degrees Celsius for 10 to 12 minutes.

Nutrition:

- Calories: 289 Fat: 15.4g Carbs: 20.5g Protein: 12.1g Fiber: 3.2g

Filled Dough Pieces In Carrot Shape

Preparation Time: 30 minutes | Cooking Time: 0 minutes | Servings: 8

Ingredients:

- 400 ml vegetable stock
- 200 g red lentils
- 1 tablespoon almond butter
- 1 pack. Pizza dough
- salt and pepper
- 1 bunch of parsley

Directions:

• Do not make funnels out of aluminum paper to hold the pizza dough in the shape of a carrot. • Roll out the dough, cut into strips and wrap around the funnels.

• Then bake at 200 degrees Celsius for about 10 minutes until they are golden brown. • In the meantime, bring the broth to a boil and cook the lentils in it.

• Season with almond butter, salt, and pepper and

let cool slightly.

- Fill the funnels with lentils and finally put a bunch of parsley on top.
- These bites go perfectly with an Easter brunch.

Nutrition:

- Calories: 229 Fat: 9.4g Carbs: 11.5g Protein: 12.1g Fiber: 3.2g

Banana Cream Stuffed Strawberries

• Preparation Time: 15-30 minutes | Cooking Time: 10 minutes | Servings: 4

Ingredients:

- 12 fresh strawberries, heads removed
- ¼ cup cashew cream
- ¼ tsp banana extract
- 1 tbsp unsweetened coconut flakes

Directions:

• Use a teaspoon to scoop out some of the strawberries pulp to create a hole within. • In a small bowl, mix the cashew cream, banana extract, and maple syrup.

• Spoon the mixture into the strawberries and garnish with the coconut flakes. Serve.

Nutrition:

• Calories 47 Fats 3. 38g Carbs 4. 11g Protein 0. 69g

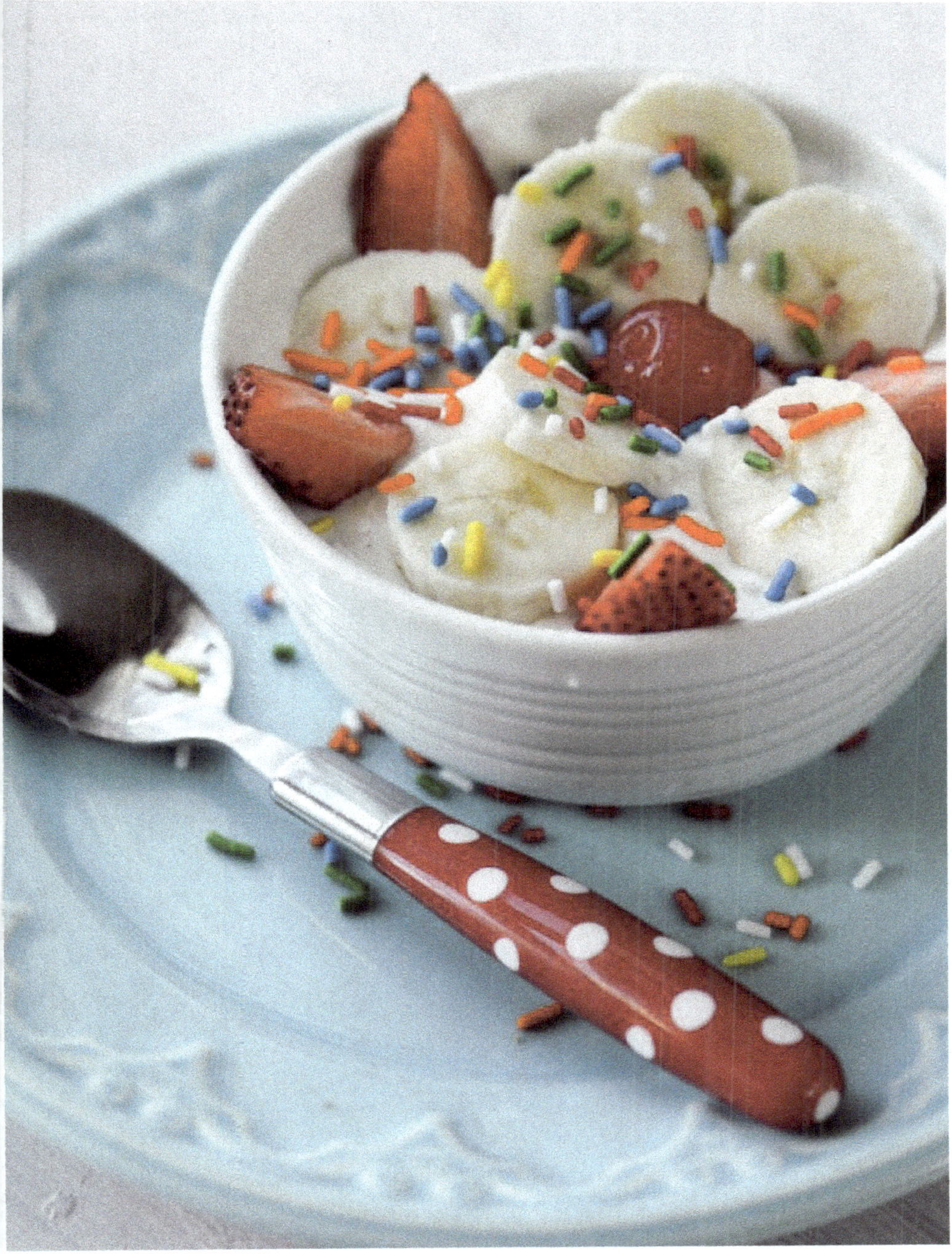

CPSIA information can be obtained
at www.ICGtesting.com
Printed in the USA
BVHW091107210621
610125BV00003B/523

9 781803 178004